T0144848

Sustaining the Caffeine Advantage

The Science of Sustained Energy,
Exercise, and Fat Burning

Jose Antonio, Ph.D., C.S.C.S., F.A.C.S.M.

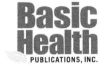

Basic
Health
PUBLICATIONS, INC.

Basic Health Publications, Inc.

Library of Congress Cataloging-in-Publication Data

Antonio Jose.
    Sustaining the caffeine advantage : the science of sustained energy, exercise, and fat burning / Jose Antonio.

    p. cm.
    Includes bibliographical references and index.
    ISBN: 978-1-59120-167-0 (Pbk.)
    ISBN: 978-1-68162-787-8 (Hardcover)

    1. Caffeine—Physiological effect. 2. Caffeine—Therapeutic use.
I. Title.

    QP801.C24A56   2005
    613.8'4—dc22

                                                    2005004576

Editor: Jane E. Morrill
Book Design and Typesetting: Gary A. Rosenberg
Cover Design: Think, Inc.

Contents

It's Not Just for Breakfast Anymore

Caffeine is the most commonly consumed supplement in the world. This is true for three primary reasons. First, it increases your mental and physical energy, enabling you to work and play longer and harder. Second, it enables you to exercise harder for a longer period of time, so you achieve your goal more quickly. Third, it helps your body to burn more fat, so you lose more weight in a shorter time.

These benefits are short-lived with traditional caffeine-delivery systems, which peak early and leave your system quickly. But times are changing. A new sustained-release caffeine delivery system is now available. Before we examine it, let's look at caffeine in general.

WHAT IS CAFFEINE?

Chemists technically refer to caffeine as an alkaloid, of which there are several types. Caffeine belongs to a specific class of alkaloids called "methylxanthines." Other members of this class include theophylline, which is used in medicines to treat asthma, and theobromine, which is found in chocolate. All methylxanthines have stimulant properties.[1]

Caffeine is chemically known as 1,3,7-trimethylxanthine. Figure 1.1 below shows its chemical structure.

The benefits of caffeine can be grouped into the following categories: energy, performance enhancement, and thermogenesis. Let's look at each of them in turn.

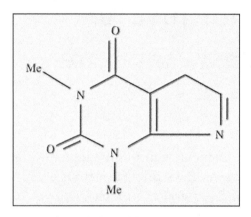

Figure 1.1
The Chemical Structure
of Caffeine
Me = methyl group CH_3
N = nitrogen
O = oxygen

Energy

Perhaps the most common reason for consuming caffeine or a caffeinated beverage is its pick-me-up effect. Let's face it. You could be moving slower than a sloth on tranquilizers, but with a little help from caffeine, you can have the energy of a race horse in the final stretch of the Kentucky Derby. Everyday experience confirms the energy benefits of caffeine, and scientists have conducted studies verifying these effects:

- It provides you with the energy to complete mental tasks faster and more easily.

- It gives you the energy to remain alert when your brain is begging for sleep.

- It furnishes the energy boost you need if you just want to feel better.

Caffeine—Yesterday and Today

Caffeine is found in more than 100 species of plants, but the most highly cultivated sources are the seeds (beans) of the berries from the coffee tree and the leaves and leaf-buds of the tea bush. Caffeine intake through coffee consumption has a long and storied history dating back to the 1400s when the Sufis of Yemen were the first to document its use.[2]

Today, caffeine is used as a morning and evening pick-me-up, a performance enhancer, and a fat-burning agent. The *Journal of the American Dietetic Association* published a recent study involving 18,081 people[3] and showed that 87 percent of them consumed food and beverages containing caffeine! The average caffeine intake was 193 milligrams (mg) of caffeine per day. As age increased, caffeine consumption also increased. Men and women aged thirty-five to sixty-four years were among the highest consumers of caffeine. The main sources of caffeine were coffee (71 percent), soft drinks (16 percent), and tea (12 percent). Coffee was the major source of caffeine in the diets of adults, whereas soft drinks were the primary source for children and teens.

One scientific study gave the subjects breakfast with either caffeinated or decaffeinated coffee. The researchers found that consuming caffeine with breakfast improved the "encoding of new information and counteracted the fatigue that developed over the test session."[4] In other words, the brain *with* caffeine was better at taking in new information and remaining alert over a period of time than it was *without* caffeine.

Another study looked at the effects of caffeine and Modafinil (a stimulant drug banned by the International Olympic Committee; IOC). It investigated the extent to which Modafinil and caffeine reversed the effects of "fatigue," defined as the decline in performance over time, during total sleep depriva-tion.[5] If you've ever stayed up all night to get that important presentation ready for an early morning meeting, you know what it's like to feel deprived of sleep.

> • • • • • **Did You Know?**
>
> Caffeine is so effective at improving exercise
> performance that the IOC at one time banned
> its use by Olympic athletes.

Investigators in this double-blind study compared the effects of 200 mg, 400 mg, and 600 mg of caffeine, 400 mg of Modafinil, and a placebo. They discovered that both 600 mg of caffeine and 400 mg of Modafinil decreased fatigue.[6] What does this tell us? That even when compared to a pharmaceu-tical drug such as Modafinil, caffeine can hold its own!

> • • • • • **Double-Blind Study**
>
> A type of study in which neither the investigators
> nor the subjects know who is taking the actual
> substance being investigated and who is taking
> the placebo, an inert substance.

Performance Enhancement

Fitness enthusiasts and Olympic athletes alike know caffeine is *the* most versatile and effective "ergogenic aid."[7-37] Whether "performance" for you means running faster, lasting longer on a treadmill, or covering more distance during a sprint, caf-feine is helpful any time you challenge your body to do more.

• • • • • **Ergogenic Aid**

A term used by exercise physiologists to denote anything an athlete can use or consume to enhance athletic performance. Typically, it refers to foods, drugs, or supplements.

What can a performance enhancer do for you on a long-term basis? Think about it. If you can last longer at your favorite exercise, you would burn more calories and, therefore, more fat. You would end up leaner, fitter, and in better shape—that's what!

David Costill, Ph.D., a prominent exercise physiologist, performed a ground-breaking study on caffeine and exercise in 1978. In this study, competitive cyclists rode until exhaustion at 80 percent of VO_2 max (maximum volume of oxygen). After consuming caffeine, the subjects were able to perform an average of ninety minutes of cycling, compared to an average of seventy-six minutes on the placebo.

The researchers also found that the subjects burned more fat on caffeine than on the placebo. Moreover, the perception of effort was much lower in the subjects who had taken caffeine, indicating that the exercise felt easier.[38] (For more information on this landmark study, see "Costill's Classic Study" in Chapter 4.)

• • • • • **VO_2 Max**

Maximal oxygen uptake (VO_2 max) is a measure of how much oxygen your body can take in and deliver to working muscles.

Thermogenesis

In thermogenesis, your body burns fats, carbohydrates, or proteins to generate heat and usable energy. The greater the thermogenic effect, the more your metabolism increases. Caffeine is thermogenic—it can stoke up your body's furnace so you burn more calories.[39–54] What's more, you burn more fat in the process. Fitness competitors often drink a strong cup of coffee or take a caffeine pill prior to exercising. That way, they can exercise harder and longer.

Thermogenesis

The technical term for the body's generation of heat and energy.

Does age make a difference in caffeine's thermogenic benefits? A recent study looked at energy expenditure, fat burning, and *norepinephrine kinetics* (how adrenaline-like hormones are metabolized) after taking caffeine or a placebo. The study used placebo-controlled double-blind conditions. The subjects were divided between older men, aged sixty-five to eighty, and younger men, aged nineteen to twenty-six, all of whom were moderate caffeine consumers.

Placebo-Controlled Study

A study that compares the effects of a "real" pill, powder, or beverage to the effects of a "fake" pill, powder, or beverage—a placebo— that looks and tastes exactly like the real one.

Caffeine consumption resulted in similar increases in caffeine levels, so both young and old subjects absorbed caffeine equally well. The metabolic rate, or energy expenditure, increased slightly more in the younger men than in the older men. According to the scientists, "older and younger men show a similar thermogenic response to caffeine ingestion." The bottom line is, caffeine significantly enhances fat burning and increases metabolic rate regardless of age.[55]

CAFFEINE'S EFFECT ON LIPOLYSIS AND OXIDATION

Caffeine has been shown to promote lipolysis. In lipolysis the body splits a fat molecule into its component parts: glycerol and free fatty acids. Then, these free fatty acids, which are liberated into the bloodstream, can be oxidized by exercising muscles and other tissues.

• • • • • Lipolysis

The technical term for how the body breaks down or splits a triglyceride or fat molecule into free fatty acids. "Lipolysis" literally means "to split fat" ("lipo" means "fat"; "lysis" means "to split").

• • • • • Oxidation

A term used by physiologists to denote the utilization of your body's fuel. When you "oxidize" fat, you burn it for fuel. The same applies to carbohydrates and protein; when you oxidize them, you burn them for fuel.

> • • • • • **Lipid Oxidation**
>
> The technical term for how your body utilizes fats (lipids) to generate energy by producing adenosine triphosphate (ATP), a process that requires oxygen.

CAFFEINE'S SAFETY

Don't be fooled by the nonsense you've heard about caffeine's being bad for your health. Caffeine not only works, it's one of the safest ingredients in existence, if used properly.

For instance, one study concluded that caffeine consumption is "*not* [emphasis added] associated with adverse effects such as general toxicity, cardiovascular effects, effects on bone status and calcium balance (with consumption of adequate calcium), changes in adult behavior, increased incidence of cancer, and effects on male fertility."[56]

The published literature provides little evidence that coffee or caffeine in typical doses increases the risk of heart attack, sudden death, or arrhythmia.[57] In fact, its beneficial effects may involve both improved insulin sensitivity and enhanced insulin response.[58] However, if you are hypertensive or have several cardiac risk factors, it would be wise for you to seek the advice of your physician before consuming caffeine.

Moreover, there is no evidence that caffeine increases the risk of cancer. Scientists found, in the Swedish Mammography Screening Cohort, that consumption of coffee, tea, and other caffeine was *not* associated with the incidence of breast cancer.[59] Furthermore, there is no evidence that caffeine has any harmful effects on bone status or calcium metabolism in individuals who ingest the recommended daily allowance of calcium.[60]

In a study of college-age women, caffeine consumption was also *not* associated with a significant reduction in rates of bone gain. Although calcium and protein nutrition affect bone gain in women in the third decade of life, moderate caffeine intake at this age—about one cup of coffee per day (103 mg)—appears to be safe for bone health.[61]

Caffeine and Pain Relief

Caffeine enhances the analgesic (pain-relieving) properties of various medications. One study looked at the effectiveness of the 100-mg diclofenac-sodium soft gel (a nonsteroidal anti-inflammatory, or NSAID) with and without 100 mg of caffeine versus a placebo in individuals during migraine attacks. The major finding of the study was that the diclofenac soft gel plus caffeine produced statistically significant benefits compared to the placebo. The diclofenac soft gel alone, however, was no better than the placebo at relieving migraine headaches.[62–64]

Another investigation looked at the benefits of acetaminophen, aspirin, and caffeine (AAC) in the treatment of severe, debilitating migraine attacks. Scientists concluded that "the nonprescription combination of AAC was well-tolerated and effective."[65] Perhaps this is one reason why caffeine helps exercise performance. You feel less pain during exercise and, therefore, can work out longer and with more intensity.

Points to Remember

Caffeine:

◆ Improves brain power and concentration.

◆ Enhances exercise performance.

◆ Increases fat burning.

◆ Raises the metabolic rate in both young and old people.

◆ Use dates back to the 1400s.

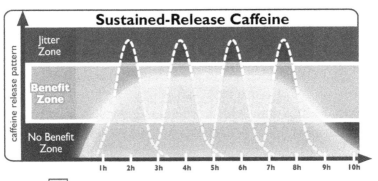

The Sustained-Release Advantage

You know what happens when you get overstimulated from consuming too much caffeine too quickly—you feel wound up, only to feel suddenly tired later in the day. Too much caffeine produces the "jitters." Too little caffeine, however, provides no therapeutic effect. What you want is a happy medium—a consistent flow of energy throughout the day. If only there were a way to consume caffeine that didn't produce the "jitters" and maintained an energy flow that lasts all day. Well, there is! (See the graph below.)

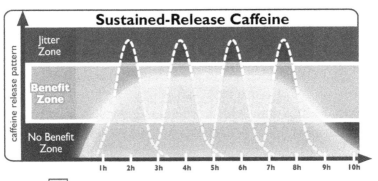

Single dose of sustained-release caffeine

Each arc represents a single dose of regular caffeine

SUSTAINED-RELEASE CAFFEINE

Sports scientists have discovered substances that, for all practical purposes, enhance performance better than whole foods do. Moreover, these scientists have scoured the globe to find safe and legal substances that actually work. They found that caffeine is the best.

Caffeine is perhaps the most thoroughly studied ingredient in the history of sports science (creatine, a muscle-building supplement, also has good scientific support). Studies have shown that caffeine can improve work output, power, and performance in both endurance and sprint-type sports. It is truly a "jack-of-all-trades" supplement.[1–5]

Like anything, however, regular caffeine isn't perfect. If you take it when you need to maintain an alert and ready state for several hours, you'll probably feel the benefits begin to wear off after a few hours. However, with *sustained*-release caffeine, the benefits would extend for a much longer period of time without crashing (see Figure 2.1). Sustained-release caffeine is superior to regular caffeine because it uses "MSR," an amazing breakthrough in delivery technology.

What Is MSR?

Matrix Sustained Release (MSR) is a technology developed to deliver consistent levels of drugs for the pharmaceutical industry. When delivering prescription drugs for which an overdose could cause toxic side effects, consistent release is especially important. Other technologies for sustained release, such as making very hard tablets, have been tried and used. Unlike these, however, MSR relies on natural binders that are attached to the active ingredient in a matrix structure and, thus, dissolve over time in the digestive tract.

The sustained, controlled disintegration of the matrix

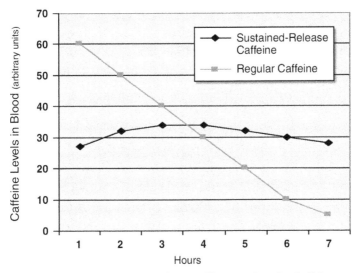

Figure 2.1 Sustained-Release Caffeine vs. Regular Caffeine

allows delivery of the active element to be fine-tuned to a specific length of time. Using this type of delivery system for caffeine extends its benefits without repeated dosing and without getting the "jitters." Numerous studies have proven this to be true. The ideal amount of time to maintain energy without interfering with sleep was considered to be eight hours, so that was the period of time chosen for the sustained release of caffeine. The authentic form of sustained-release caffeine using the MSR delivery system that has proven effective in scientific research has been patented to protect products based on MSR from imitators selling inferior products. To get all the benefits of sustained-release caffeine, look for patent number 5,744,164.[6]

Be Alert!

Numerous investigations have been conducted into the benefits of caffeine. The April 2000 issue of *Human Psychopharma-*

cology discusses the pharmacodynamic (reactions between drugs and living beings) profile of a single oral dose of 600 milligrams (mg) of the patented MSR form of caffeine. This is the authentic form of sustained-release caffeine that has proven effective in scientific research.

One study looked at thirty-six-hour sleep deprivation using a classic, randomized, double-blind, placebo-controlled study design. Sustained-release caffeine significantly reduced the harmful effects of sleep deprivation, as shown on an electroencephalogram (EEG), and improved psychomotor performance. The effect peaked in four hours and was maintained until the end of sleep deprivation twenty-four hours later (see Figure 2.2). This study shows that a single dose of sustained-release caffeine possesses "alerting effects which are able to reverse the deleterious effect of thirty-six hours of sleep deprivation for at least twenty-four hours."[7]

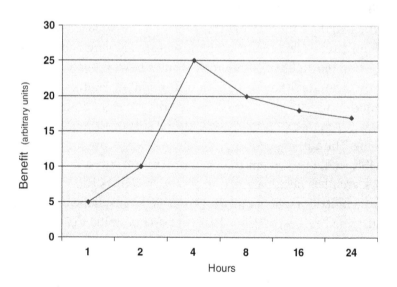

Figure 2.2   Longevity of Sustained-Release Caffeine (600-mg dosage)

•••••Randomized Study

A study in which the subjects are divided into two or more equal groups and are randomly assigned to one of the groups. Neither the investigators conducting the study nor the subjects involved choose who goes into which group.

There is more proof that sustained-release caffeine works in the *Journal of Sleep Research.* Investigators looked at the effects of sustained-release caffeine (daily dose of 600 mg) on alertness and cognitive performance during sixty-four hours of continuous wakefulness in a double-blind, randomized, placebo-controlled, two-way crossover study. A dose of 300 mg of sustained-release caffeine or placebo was given twice a day during the sleep-deprivation period. (If you think you see a pattern, you're correct. The favored dose in these investigations seems to be 300–600 mg/day.)

•••••Crossover Study

A study in which each subject, in essence, gets both the real pill and the placebo pill. For example, in testing whether a caffeine pill aids exercise endurance, a subject might take the placebo and then perform the exercise test. A week later, the subject would take the real pill and then perform the exercise test. The order in which a subject is tested (placebo or real pill, first or second) is random.

Alertness was objectively assessed with continuous EEG monitoring and standard psychological tests. The cognitive functions of information processing and working memory were further assessed. Not surprisingly, the subjects taking sustained-release caffeine were more alert from beginning to end of sleep deprivation. In fact, some cognitive functions actually improved during the sleep-deprivation period. The conclusion was that 300 mg of sustained-release caffeine given twice daily during sixty-four hours of sleep deprivation lessened the impairment of vigilance and cognitive functions.[8] In other words, if you take two 300-mg doses per day of sustained-release caffeine over a period of prolonged wakefulness, you'll be more alert and aware and more likely to use better judgment. (There's more on sleep deprivation in the next chapter.)

Jet Lag, Anyone?

The body has an internal time clock, of sorts, that is set for a sleep-wake cycle. If you've traveled across several time zones, you know what a killer jet lag can be. You don't know if it's morning or afternoon, breakfast or dinner. Overall, you feel tired and miserable, and you wish you were home. Sustained-release caffeine might be the solution to your jet lag–induced problems.

In an intriguing study, a group of U.S. Air Force reservists received either sustained-release caffeine (300 mg), melatonin (5 mg), or a placebo before, during, and after an around-the-world flight. Researchers found that both caffeine and melatonin negated the rise in cortisol that occurs during transcontinental flights. In other words, the body has less of a "stress" response with caffeine than without it. Both sustained-release caffeine and melatonin also resynchronized hormone rhythms more quickly during the four days following a flight with a seven-hour time loss.[9] So, if you're going from New York to Las Vegas, you might want to drink an espresso or two to maximize your gambling and partying activities—unless, of course, you have sustained-release caffeine handy.

• • • • • Melatonin

A hormone secreted by the brain that helps regulate sleep-wake cycles.

• • • • • Cortisol

Also known as the "stress hormone." Cortisol levels rise when the body is being subjected to internal or external stressors.

PURE ENERGY

It's as clear as the ocean in Fiji that sustained-release caffeine helps brain function if you're sleep-deprived or flying from Paris to New York. But sustained-release caffeine has another trick up its sleeve: It aids fat loss. As you've learned, caffeine stimulates lipolysis (breaking down of fat), energy expenditure (burning more calories), and lipid oxidation (the burning of fat). *The American Journal of Clinical Nutrition* reported on a study that compared whether caffeine or a placebo metabolized more fat. The caffeine used was half regular caffeine and half sustained-release caffeine.

By the last hour of the test, the caffeine subjects were

metabolizing twice as much fat as those on the placebo, and the average metabolic rate rose 13.3 percent (see Figure 2.3). Interestingly enough, after consuming caffeine, the rate of fat burning increased 44 percent—*even while sitting still*—whereas the amount of fat burned increased 2.3-fold. In other words, consuming caffeine dramatically raises the energy expended and promotes fat burning (see Figure 2.4).[10] Add exercise to this prescription, and imagine how much fat you'd burn!

CLEAR EVIDENCE

Sustained-release caffeine clearly works. Not only does it dramatically reduce the negative effects of sleep deprivation, it also decreases cortisol levels and promotes a significant increase in metabolic rate and fat oxidation. With a sustained-release delivery system, you get all the benefits of caffeine without the "crash and burn" of overstimulation.

Points to Remember

Sustained-release caffeine has:

◆ A pharmaceutical-style delivery system.

◆ Smooth effects.

◆ Longer effects than regular caffeine.

◆ No "jitters" or overstimulation.

◆ Requires just a single dose with no need for multiple dosing.

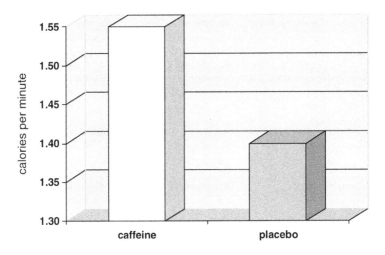

Figure 2.3   Caffeine Increased Energy Expenditure[11]
The dosage was 5 milligrams per kilogram (mg/kg) of sustained-release caffeine and 5 mg/kg of regular caffeine

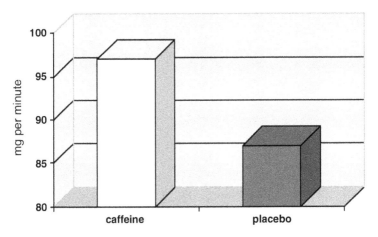

Figure 2.4   Caffeine Increased Fat Burning

Energize Me!

affeine epitomizes energy. In fact, for either mental or physical activity, there isn't a better or safer energizer anywhere. Since the most common cause of fatigue or *malaise* is no sleep, what better time could there be to test the effects of caffeine than during sleep deprivation?

SLEEP DEPRIVATION

As you've probably guessed from reading the previous chapter, sleep deprivation is widely used as a basis for testing the effectiveness of caffeine. One study looked at the reductions in cognitive and physical performance caused by lack of sleep. Activities were chosen to simulate "the physical challenges that might occur during a military scenario involving a period of sleep loss."[1] Indeed, what could be more stressful than being in a battle, knowing that if you fall asleep, you might never wake up? That's a situation where you have to perform, even if you haven't slept for days.

This study was a double-blind caffeine and placebo trial involving a control day and sleep period followed by twenty-eight hours without sleep. The subjects were given 400 milligrams (mg) of caffeine, after which they began a two-hour forced march followed by a sandbag-piling task. Five-and-a-half hours later, the subjects were given two 100-mg doses of caffeine at two-hour increments. Two hours after the final dose of caffeine, the subjects ran a treadmill to exhaustion at 85 percent of maximal aerobic power, or VO_2 max (maximum volume of oxygen).

What did the researchers find? First, they discovered that caffeine had no effect on heart rate or oxygen consumption, but it did decrease what scientists call "ratings of perceived exertion (RPE)." In other words, the exercise the subjects performed didn't feel as hard with caffeine. Furthermore, the amount of time required to complete the sandbag-piling task was 6.5 percent less with caffeine than it was with the placebo (see Figure 3.1).

Time to exhaustion on the treadmill increased significantly

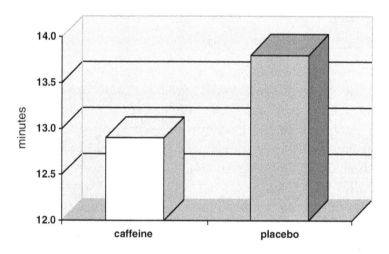

Figure 3.1   Caffeine Improved Sandbag-Piling Performance

(by 25 percent) with caffeine, compared to placebo. The scientists concluded "that caffeine is an effective strategy to maintain physical performance during an overnight period of sleep loss at levels comparable to the rested state."[2]

Help for the Weary

In another randomized, double-blind, crossover, placebo-controlled study, investigators looked at the pharmacodynamic (reactions between drugs and living beings) profile of a single oral dose of 600 mg of the patented form of sustained-release caffeine. The subjects were kept awake for thirty-six hours and were studied using an electroencephalogram (EEG) and various measures of psychomotor and cognitive processes that tested brain function.

Caffeine significantly counteracted the detrimental effects of sleep deprivation. In other words, if you're feeling weary because you haven't had enough sleep, caffeine can help increase your alertness. The sustained-release caffeine effect peaked four hours after dosing and was maintained until the end of sleep deprivation, twenty-four hours after dosing. The results demonstrate that a single dose of sustained-release caffeine has alerting effects that can turn back the harmful effects of thirty-six hours of sleep deprivation to some degree for at least twenty-four hours.[3] The bottom line is: Caffeine improves brain function, and the effects of a single dose of caffeine can, indeed, last a full day!

Another study found that 300 mg of sustained-release caffeine given twice daily during a sixty-four-hour period of sleep deprivation counteracts the damage to vigilance and cognitive functions.[4] In other words, caffeine alleviates any normal sleep-deprivation problems you might suffer.

Morning Get Up and Go

In addition to the soldier in action or the sleep-deprived college student cramming for exams, caffeine can help *you* perk up after a normal night's rest. Like many Americans, when you wake up, the first thing you probably do is drag yourself to the coffeepot and brew some caffeine-rich coffee. And if you follow your mom's advice, you never skip breakfast! What happens when you combine breakfast and caffeine?

One study looked at subjects randomly assigned to receive breakfast (cereal) and a caffeinated or decaffeinated beverage, or no breakfast with a caffeinated or decaffeinated beverage. The results showed that those who consumed breakfast cereal had a more positive mood at the start of the test session, performed better on a spatial-memory task, and felt calmer at the end of the test session than those in the no-breakfast category. Consuming caffeine improved the "encoding of new information and counteracted the fatigue that developed over the test session."[5] So, if you want to perform at your peak during that morning exam or business meeting, you should definitely eat breakfast and consume some caffeine.

Investigations have shown that caffeine improves mental performance, makes you more alert, and improves your feelings of well-being. Even the military has found that caffeine is an aid for soldiers who are excessively sleep-deprived. Their studies indicate that even the "cognitive component of the shooting task (that is, target detection) can benefit from caffeine."[6]

MOOD AND PSYCHOMOTOR SKILLS

Scientists in one study took moderate caffeine consumers and deprived them of caffeine overnight. They were then given one of four treatments: all placebo, all caffeine, caffeine-placebo-placebo, or caffeine-caffeine-placebo, where the amount of caffeine in each instance was similar to that in a cup of home-brewed coffee (about 103 mg).

Caffeine or a placebo was administered double-blind in a fruit-juice drink. Before and after drinking the juice, the participants completed a mood questionnaire and psychomotor performance tests. When caffeine was delivered, there was a significant increase in energy and improvement in psychomotor performance compared to the placebo.[7]

SLEEP-RELATED ACCIDENTS

Imagine driving from New York to Key West. You suddenly realize that Florida is one *very* long state. I-95 starts to look like a big blur, and your brain is begging for sleep. With eighteen-wheelers whizzing by you at the speed of sound, falling asleep at the wheel is not an option. What can you do?

Scientists have found that sleep-related vehicle accidents are most common early in the morning, especially with younger drivers. In two independent studies following a night of either restricted sleep or none at all, experienced young drivers were given 200 mg of caffeine (equivalent to about two cups of coffee) versus placebo. Then, they drove continuously for two hours in an immobile car on an interactive, computer-generated, dull, monotonous roadway. (Just thinking about it makes me tired.) Driving incidents such as lane drifting, sleepiness, and brain activity occurred.

In the first study, the subjects were given five hours of sleep before the test. Caffeine significantly reduced driving incidents and subjective sleepiness throughout the two-hour drive. In the second study, the subjects were not given any sleep prior to the test. In this case, sleepiness profoundly affected all measurements, and driving was terminated after one hour.

Caffeine reduced driving incidents significantly over the first thirty minutes and subjective sleepiness for an hour. Even after no sleep at all, caffeine had a positive effect on psycho-motor performance and energy.[8]

Imagine you could take sustained-release caffeine before a long-distance drive. You'd be alert but not overstimulated. You'd have no problem driving for several hours, and you wouldn't experience a mental "crash." Instead, you'd get to your destination more quickly and get extra rest and relaxation there.

BRAIN FOOD

The relationship between habitual coffee and tea consumption and cognitive performance was examined using data from a cross-section of 9,003 British adults in the Health and Lifestyle Survey. It found, in essence, the more coffee with caffeine the subjects drank, the better they did on brain-function tests.[9] That's something to chew on.

Points to Remember

Caffeine:

* Improves performance on tasks that require sustained attention.

* Produces improvement on tasks needing logical reasoning.

* Increases achievement on tasks requiring semantic memory.

* Enhances the absorption of new information.

- Increases the ability to remain alert over a period of time.

- Counteracts the harmful effects of sleep deprivation, as shown on an EEG.

- Improves performance of motor actions coming directly from mental activity.

- Increases performance and speed of reaction on a variety of brain-function tests.

- Significantly decreases bodily sway due to fatigue.

- Enhances overall alertness and mental function.

- Decreases the inconsistencies in knowledge that accompany sleep deprivation.

Peak Performance

N umerous studies show that caffeine improves exercise performance.[1–25] In fact, caffeine is such a great performance enhancer that at one time the International Olympic Committee (IOC) banned its use by Olympic athletes. They have since lifted the ban, so if you want to run longer, pedal faster, or swim harder, there is no better supplement.

COSTILL'S CLASSIC STUDY

Dr. David Costill, one of the preeminent exercise physiologists of the twentieth century, was the first to show the ergogenic effects of caffeine in his simple but elegant study. To determine the effects caffeine consumption has on metabolism and performance during prolonged exercise, a group of competitive cyclists exercised until exhaustion on a bicycle "ergometer" at 80 percent of VO_2 max (maximum volume of oxygen). One test was performed an hour after ingesting decaffeinated coffee, while a second test was carried out after consuming coffee containing 330 milligrams (mg) of caffeine. The caffeine group cycled for ninety minutes, versus seventy-six minutes for the decaffeinated group (see Figure 4.1).

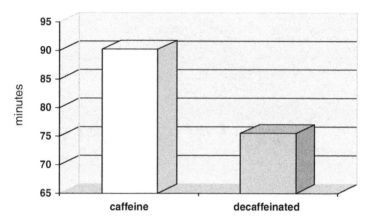

Figure 4.1   Caffeine Lengthened Cycling Time

> • • • • • **Ergometer**
>
> An instrument that measures the amount of
> work that a muscle or group of muscles does.

The group that consumed caffeine also burned more fat. Calculations of carbohydrate metabolism from respiratory exchange ratio (RER) data revealed that the subjects burned roughly the same amount of carbohydrates in both trials. However, the group that drank caffeinated coffee burned much more fat than the group that drank the decaffeinated coffee (see Figure 4.2).

Another interesting finding was that exercise "felt" easier after caffeinated coffee than after decaffeinated. To summarize this seminal study: Caffeine helps you exercise longer; the exercise feels easier; and you burn more fat.[26]

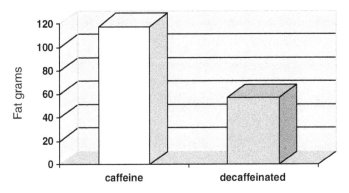

Figure 4.2   Caffeine Resulted in Significantly More Fat Burned

ENDURANCE SPORTS

Ever since Costill's study, there has been an abundance of research on caffeine and performance. Caffeine can improve how long you last on a treadmill; it can enhance your sprint-swimming performance; and it increases endurance in a variety of other activities, such as cycling. Here's the proof.

In a study similar to Costill's, the subjects cycled to exhaustion at approximately 80 percent of VO_2 max after ingesting a placebo or the equivalent of about seven cups of caffeinated coffee. In this study, as in Costill's, the caffeine-consuming subjects cycled ninety minutes, versus seventy-six minutes for the placebo. During the first fifteen minutes of exercise, the caffeine group used significantly less glycogen (carbohydrates stored in muscle) than the placebo group. This "spared glycogen" was available later in the exercise period and contributed to the longer time to exhaustion.

According to the authors, increased utilization of fat after consuming caffeine "may inhibit carbohydrate use at rest and early during exercise. . . . In other words, you can spare a bit of your stored muscle glycogen . . . while burning more [of the] fat that's stored in your muscles, as well as in your blood, as a result of caffeine consumption!"[27]

●●●●● **Effective Dose**

A dose of caffeine useful for performance enhancement lies in the range of at least 250–350 mg.

Rise and Shine

Want to run longer or cycle farther? If you took a dose of caffeine in the morning, would you need to take another dose in the afternoon to maintain an ergogenic effect? In one study, the subjects performed exercise rides to exhaustion at 80 percent of VO_2 max one hour after consuming a placebo, 175 mg of caffeine (low), or 350 mg of caffeine (high).

Two exercise rides were performed weekly on the same day, once in the morning and five hours later in the afternoon under four sets of circumstances: A) high caffeine in the morning, low caffeine in the afternoon; B) placebo both morning and afternoon; C) high caffeine in the morning, placebo in the afternoon; and D) placebo in the morning, high caffeine in the afternoon.

Caffeine increased exercise time to exhaustion in the morning (see Figure 4.3). This effect was maintained in the afternoon and was greater than the placebo regardless of whether caffeine or the placebo followed the initial morning dose. Caffeine dosing in the afternoon also increased the amount of time to exhaustion when it was given after the placebo in the morning (see Figure 4.4). Investigators concluded that redosing with caffeine after exhaustive morning exercise was not necessary to maintain the ergogenic effect during subsequent exercise six hours later.[28]

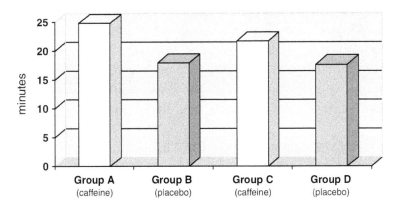

Figure 4.3   Caffeine Improved Morning Performance
Both caffeine groups (A and C) performed significantly better than the placebo groups.

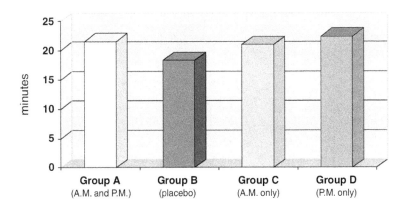

Figure 4.4   Caffeine Improved Afternoon Performance
Group C took caffeine in the morning only, yet maintained good performance in the afternoon. Group A took caffeine in the morning and afternoon, whereas Group D took caffeine in the afternoon only.

The moral of the story is that caffeine works in the morning and in the afternoon. For exercise performance, a single dose of approximately 300–400 mg of caffeine in the morning can maintain an ergogenic effect throughout the day. (The placebos had no effect on performance.)

The evidence is overwhelming that caffeine can boost endurance. Many scientists conclude that enhanced endurance may result in part from spared muscle glycogen, increased lipolysis and fat oxidation, a decrease in pain sensation, and a profound effect on the central nervous system.[29]

SPEED/STRENGTH SPORTS

Does caffeine help the "big" guys in speed/strength sports, as well? In a word, yes! For example, maximal *anaerobic* power (maximum attainable pace or effort) increased significantly after the subjects ingested less than three cups of caffeinated coffee (see Figure 4.5).

The subjects in one study were tested to determine the effect of caffeine on the strength and power of knee extensors

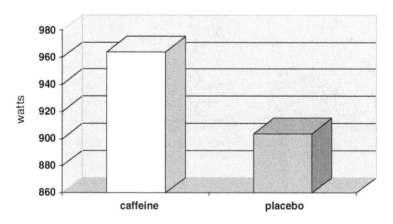

Figure 4.5　Caffeine Improved Anaerobic Power

and flexors (the quadriceps and hamstring muscles). The caffeine dose was equivalent to seven or more cups of coffee. Muscular power was measured at slow, medium, and fast speeds of movement. The study found significant caffeine-related increases in extensor torque and flexor torque at both fast and slow speeds. No significant effects were found in any variable for the placebo trial. According to the authors, "It was concluded that caffeine can favorably affect some strength parameters in highly resistance-trained males."[30]

Subjects in another study swam 100 meters freestyle at maximum speed twice—once after consuming about two cups of caffeinated coffee, and once after a placebo. Only the trained athletes swam faster during the caffeine trial. This is further evidence that caffeine isn't just for endurance athletes.[31]

PAIN NO MORE

Many over-the-counter pain medications have caffeine added to them because enhancing aspirin and acetaminophen products with caffeine makes them relieve headache pain about 40 percent better. Caffeine also helps the body absorb these medications better, allowing you to get back to your daily life more quickly.[32]

Besides headaches, pain management can play a significant role in exercise, too. Whether you're on the treadmill or bench-pressing multiple sets and repetitions, sometimes you just don't have the pain tolerance to push yourself.

Believe it or not, this may be one of the reasons why caffeine works so well. A study of low caffeine–consuming college-age subjects compared the effects of low caffeine, high caffeine, and placebo on thirty minutes of moderate-intensity cycling exercise (to 60 percent of VO_2 peak). The caffeine increased blood pressure in a dose-dependent fashion, but these blood-pressure effects were not maintained during exercise. In leg-

●●●●●● Caffeine Effectiveness
    ●   After Creatine Loading
    ●
    ●   If you're a creatine and caffeine consumer, you
    ●   should know caffeine is effective regardless of
           whether you take creatine or not. According to
           a recent study, "Acute caffeine ingestion was
           found to be ergogenic after six days of creatine
           supplementation and caffeine abstinence."[33]

muscle pain ratings, the higher the dose of caffeine was, the more pain relief it provided (see Figure 4.6). According to the authors, "The results support the conclusion that caffeine ingestion has a dose-response effect on reducing leg-muscle pain during exercise, and that these effects do not depend on caffeine-induced increases in systolic blood pressure during exercise."[34]

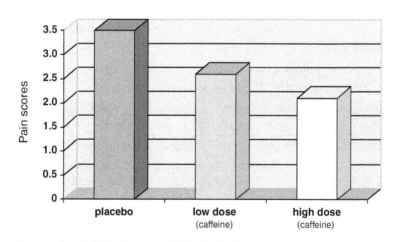

Figure 4.6   Caffeine Decreased Pain During Exercise
The lower the pain perception number, the greater the amount of pain relief.

HOW DOES CAFFEINE WORK?

The precise mechanism by which caffeine enhances performance in the body is not entirely known. There are several theories, however, that might explain it.

For one, caffeine increases muscle-contraction force during low-frequency stimulation (a form of electrical muscle agitation) by activating the release of calcium from the *sarcoplasmic reticulum* (a structure in muscle that stores and releases the calcium needed to produce a muscle contraction).

Studies have shown that caffeine enhances fat burning and spares glycogen (stored carbohydrates). That's another possible explanation. A group of Canadian scientists confirmed that the "ergogenic effect of caffeine in endurance-exercise performance occurs directly at the skeletal muscle level."[35]

Either way, as scientists unravel the exact nature of caffeine's effects, athletes and fitness enthusiasts already know beyond a shadow of a doubt that it works. Period!

Points to Remember

Caffeine:

- Improves endurance during cycling.
- Adds to the pace or effort attainable during exercise.
- Improves muscle strength.
- Lengthens the time to exhaustion.
- Increases the speed possible when swimming sprints.
- Directly affects muscle fibers.
- WORKS!

Fat Assassin

I f you want to burn more fat, look no further. Caffeine is your best friend in the fight against an expanding waistline. Some of the best physique competitors take caffeine pills or drink massive quantities of coffee prior to exercising in order to burn fat. This tactic is especially good in the morning.

When you first wake up in the morning, your body is oxidizing or burning primarily fat calories. As soon as you consume a mixed meal (that is, a mixture of carbohydrates, protein, and fat), your body shifts its metabolic gear and starts burning more carbohydrates and less fat. Why? Because it's easier for your body to burn sugars.

If you want to stay in fat-burning mode, consume caffeine or coffee (without sugar). In addition to burning fat, the added caffeine further promotes lipolysis and lipid oxidation, so your exercising muscles will use the liberated free fatty acids from lipolysis as a fuel source.

BURN, BABY, BURN!

The thermogenic effect of caffeine is undeniable. An abundance of data shows the magnificent fat-burning, metabolism-enhancing effects of caffeine. For instance, a single dose of 100 milligrams (mg) of caffeine (the amount in about one cup of coffee) increased the resting metabolic rate (RMR) of both lean and post-obese volunteers by 3 to 4 percent over two and a half hours. The caffeine also improved what researchers called the "defective diet–induced thermogenesis observed in the post-obese subjects."

Furthermore, repeated caffeine administration over a twelve-hour day increased the energy expenditure and calorie consumption of both groups during that period. For example, if you assume the "average" increase to be 100 calories burned seven days a week for a year, that could theoretically result in a twelve-pound weight loss. The authors of this study concluded that "caffeine at commonly consumed doses can have a significant influence on energy balance and may promote thermogenesis in the treatment of obesity."[1] In other words, you will burn more calories all day long if you consume caffeine.

Couch Potato versus Athlete

What would happen if you were to consume an ascending dose of caffeine (for example, 100 mg, 200 mg, 400 mg)? According to one study, caffeine increased energy expenditure in a dose-dependent manner: In other words, the more you take, the greater the response is.[2] Anyone who drinks espresso can vouch for that!

One study compared the caffeine response in endurance-trained subjects to that in sedentary subjects. The test subjects were also classified into regular and nonregular caffeine consumers. Before taking caffeine, no significant metabolic differences among the groups were observed. However, caffeine consumption resulted in a greater RMR increase in the inactive subjects than in the exercise-trained subjects. Whether a test subject was a regular or nonregular caffeine consumer did not appear to be significant. No other differences were observed between exercise-trained and inactive subjects.[3]

You can glean several important pieces of information from this study. First, caffeine consumption does not have a negative effect on blood pressure or heart rate, and clearly, it elevates metabolic rate. Yet, in those who are endurance-trained, the response seems to be blunted. This doesn't mean that everyone who exercises will get a smaller thermogenic effect. It makes sense that endurance-trained individuals, who tend to be smaller and lighter, would have a lesser response. The endurance-trained body tries to conserve what little body mass (and muscle mass) it has. An enormous thermogenic response to a caffeine challenge wouldn't make sense. Moreover, couch potatoes may derive greater benefits from caffeine than their endurance-trained brethren. This bodes well for those looking for a practical weight-loss solution.

> ● ● ● ● ● ● **Good News About Weighty Matters**
>
> One study concluded, "caffeine at commonly consumed doses can have a significant influence on energy balance and may promote thermogenesis in the treatment of obesity."[4]

Young and Restless

We know that older individuals *absorb* caffeine as well as younger people do (see Chapter 1), but does caffeine *burn fat* as well in young and old? Yes, it does. Caffeine consumption by both young and old resulted in similar increases in energy expenditure (see Figure 5.1), so reaping the benefits of caffeine doesn't diminish as age increases.[5]

In another study, subjects consumed decaffeinated coffee with or without 200 mg of added caffeine. RMR was measured in the fasting state and up to three hours after consuming coffee. The metabolic rate increased by 7 percent during the three hours of examination. These results are similar to the previous study's and suggest a dose/response relationship between caffeine consumption and RMR.[6]

Another group of subjects received caffeine in much higher doses and were studied for 90 minutes before and 240 minutes after ingestion. The average thermic effect was 13.3 percent. Caffeine also doubled the turnover of lipids and raised the fat burned by 44 percent for the study subjects who were sitting still (more fat would have been burned with even moderate exercise). Clearly, caffeine has some very potent effects on metabolism and the turnover of your body's fat stores.[7]

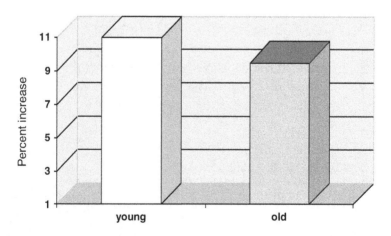

Figure 5.1   Caffeine Elevated Metabolism in Both Young and Old Subjects

A Lean Mean Machine

Caffeine gives a thermogenic boost to young and old alike, although lean endurance athletes may not have as great a response. What about lean versus obese individuals? In a head-to-head comparison, lean and obese subjects were studied in a respiratory chamber after coffee consumption. On one occasion, subjects consumed caffeinated coffee and on the other, decaffeinated. In terms of total caffeine for the day, they ingested 20 mg/kg of body weight or about 1,200 mg for a 132-pound woman. Wow! That dose would wake the planet Jupiter! The results revealed that the metabolic rate increase was less in obese than in lean subjects, but both fat and carbohydrate oxidation were enhanced after consuming caffeine.[8]

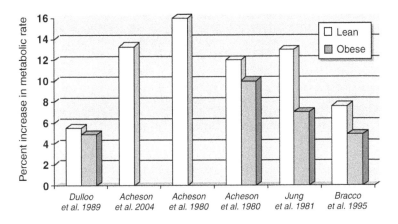

Figure 5.2   Metabolic Increases with Caffeine for Lean vs. Obese

The effects on thermogenesis are dose- and time-dependent. The Dulloo, et al. (1989) study measured twenty-four-hour energy expenditure after giving 100 mg of caffeine every two hours for twelve hours. The two Acheson, et al. (1980) studies provided a lower (4 mg/kg) and higher (8 mg/kg) single dose and measured RMR for two and a half hours. Acheson's later work (2004) provided 10 mg/kg dose in a 50/50 mix of regular and the patented MSR form of sustained-release caffeine and examined a four-hour response after caffeine ingestion. The Jung, et al. (1981) study gave a 4 mg/kg single dose and measured RMR for two hours. Finally, the Bracco, et al. (1995) study measured twenty-four-hour energy expenditure after giving a 4 mg/kg dose *five times* over an entire day.[9–11] Thus, even though the total thermogenic effect is lower in the Bracco study, keep in mind that Acheson measured it only for a few hours. If Acheson had carried the measurements for twenty-four hours, you'd see a much lower average increase in RMR. Nonetheless, it's clear when you look at acute (a few hours) and long-term (a full day) response to caffeine ingestion, you can significantly elevate RMR—from 5 to 15 percent, give or take.

Points to Remember

Caffeine:

- Increases the body's ability to produce energy by 5 to 15 percent.

- Improves fat burning.

- Raises the metabolic rate in young and old people.

- Elevates metabolism in both lean and obese individuals.

- Has a greater effect at higher doses.

- Further enhances fat burning when taken before exercise.

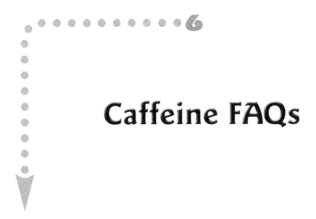

Caffeine FAQs

WHAT IS CAFFEINE?

Caffeine belongs to a specific class of alkaloids called "methyl-xanthines." Its chemical structure is shown in Figure 1.1 on page 2. Other members of this class are found in medicines that treat asthma and in chocolate.

WHAT DOES CAFFEINE TASTE LIKE?

Caffeine has a bitter taste.

WHAT IS A "MODERATE" INTAKE OF CAFFEINE?

Approximately 300 milligrams (mg) a day is considered a moderate intake of caffeine for an adult. That's roughly three cups of brewed coffee.

WHY IS CAFFEINE ADDED TO SO MANY MEDICINES?

Caffeine enhances the pain-relieving properties of medications. In a study of migraine patients, a non-steroidal anti-inflammatory (NSAID) with caffeine produced statistically significant benefits over the NSAID alone or placebo.[1-3]

Another investigation of migraine patients found that "the nonprescription combination of [acetaminophen, aspirin, and caffeine] AAC was well-tolerated and effective."[4]

Is caffeine banned by any sport-governing bodies?

Caffeine was banned by the International Olympic Committee (IOC) at one time, but it is no longer banned by any sport-governing body, including the National Collegiate Athletic Association (NCAA), the National Football League (NFL), Major League Baseball (MLB), and the National Basketball Association (NBA).

What dosage of caffeine is effective to enhance exercise performance?

Somewhere in the range of 250–350 mg of caffeine seems to be enough to induce a performance-enhancing effect.

How much caffeine is needed to improve mental alertness and energy?

A range of 300–600 mg caffeine is effective for enhancing energy.

What about fat burning—how much caffeine is needed for that?

A range of 280–560 mg will stoke your metabolic furnace.

Can you overdose on caffeine?

There are case reports of caffeine toxicity from an overdose. For instance, one individual consumed approximately 3,570 mg of caffeine in a suicide attempt and developed *rhabdomyolysis* (the release of muscle-fiber contents into circulation) and acute kidney failure. The patient was treated successfully. According to doctors, this case "represents a rarely reported complication of caffeine intoxication, *rhabdomyolysis*, which occurred in the absence of other toxins or conditions that predispose to muscle necrosis."[5]

In another case a twenty-year-old bulimic woman ingested 20,000 mg of caffeine in a suicide attempt. After being evaluated and discharged from the emergency room, she was readmitted with electrocardiogram (ECG) changes and was ultimately found to have suffered a subendocardial infarction (a type of heart attack). Keep in mind that these doses are massively greater than a typical daily serving of caffeine. To put this into perspective, the amount of caffeine is equivalent to 78 diet sodas and 438 diet sodas in the first and second cases, respectively. A lethal dosage of caffeine, which is reported to kill 50 percent of the population, is estimated by some to be 10,000 mg taken orally; that's equivalent to 167 cups of tea.[6]

SHOULD PREGNANT WOMEN AVOID CAFFEINE?

One study suggests that caffeine consumption may produce a small decrease in birth weight; however, it is "unlikely to be clinically important" except for women consuming 600 mg or more of caffeine per day.[7] Another study looked at caffeine intake among mothers of small-for-gestational-age (SGA) infants, compared to that among mothers of non-SGA infants. The mothers of SGA infants drank more caffeine in the third trimester than the mothers of non-SGA infants. Scientists concluded that "high caffeine intake in the third trimester may be a risk factor for fetal growth retardation, in particular if the fetus is a boy."[8] Also, high intake of caffeine prior to pregnancy seems to be associated with an increased risk of spontaneous abortion.[9] The prudent course of action would be to limit caffeine consumption to less than 200 mg daily if you're planning to get pregnant. Women who are pregnant should seek their physician's advice.

What is the effect of caffeine on children?

Generally, caffeine is well-tolerated in usual dietary amounts. Individuals differ in their susceptibility to caffeine-related adverse effects, which in turn may influence their caffeine consumption. Overall, the effects of caffeine in children seem to be modest and typically innocuous.[10]

However, like any substance, there is a potential for abuse. One study reported on children and adolescents who have daily or near-daily headaches and excessive consumption of caffeine in the form of cola drinks; that's a minimum of 192.88 mg of caffeine daily, and an average of 1,414.5 mg of caffeine a week (in the range of 1,350–2,700 mg). Subjects were encouraged to gradually withdraw from cola drinks, which led to a complete cessation of all headaches in most of them, while a few continued to suffer from headaches.[11] Based on available evidence, scientists have concluded that a 100-pound child could consume 113 mg of caffeine, or about two-thirds of one cola drink, without objectionable effects.[12]

Is caffeine addictive?

Believe it or not, this isn't a trick question. Some people liken caffeine "addiction" to a shopping "addiction" or TV "addiction." However, caffeine is not addictive by accepted definitions in the neuroscience literature. When regular caffeine consumption is abruptly ceased, some individuals may experience headache, fatigue, or drowsiness, but is this an "addiction" in the strictest sense? According to a study published in the journal *Brain Research*, "low doses of caffeine which reflect the usual human level of consumption fail to activate reward circuits in the brain, and thus provide functional evidence of the very low addictive potential of caffeine."[13]

CAN CAFFEINE INCREASE THE RISK OF HEART DISEASE?

Contrary to popular belief, there is little evidence in the published literature that coffee/caffeine in typical dosages increases the risk of heart attack, sudden death, or arrhythmia.[14] In one of the largest studies ever conducted, The Nurses' Health Study and Health Professionals' Follow-up Study, scientists followed 41,934 men from 1986 to 1998 and 84,276 women from 1980 to 1998. These participants did not have diabetes, cancer, or cardiovascular disease at the beginning of the study. Coffee consumption was assessed every two to four years through validated questionnaires. What did the scientists discover?

Scientists discovered an inverse association between coffee intake and type 2 diabetes after adjustments for age, body mass index (BMI), and other risk factors. Also, long-term total caffeine intake from coffee and other sources was associated with a statistically significant *lower* risk for diabetes in both men and women.[15] In plain English, this means that coffee/caffeine consumption may in fact be good for you!

Another study indicated that high consumers of coffee have a reduced risk of type 2 diabetes and impaired glucose tolerance. Beneficial effects may involve both improved insulin sensitivity and enhanced insulin response.[16] However, if you are hypertensive or have several cardiac risk factors, you should check with your physician.

DOES CAFFEINE CAUSE CANCER?

There is no evidence that caffeine increases your risk of cancer. In the Swedish Mammography Screening Cohort, comprised of 59,036 women, scientists found that consumption of coffee, tea, and other caffeine was not associated with the incidence of breast cancer.[17] In a much smaller case/control comparison of women with and without benign breast disease, no differences were found in coffee and tea consumption patterns.[18] Even high-risk mice given caffeine showed an inhibition of tumor formation.[19]

DOES CAFFEINE AFFECT BONE-MINERAL CONTENT IN WOMEN?

Not if you add 1–2 tablespoons of milk to your coffee! Low calcium intake, per se, is the main culprit, not the consumption of caffeinated beverages. The negative effect of caffeine on calcium absorption is small enough to be fully offset by as little as 1–2 tablespoons of milk per cup, according to a study published in 2002.[20] There is *no* evidence that caffeine has any harmful effect on bone status or on calcium economy in individuals who consume the recommended daily allowance of calcium.[21]

In a study of college-age women, caffeine consumption was found *not* to be associated with a significant reduction in the rate of bone gain. Although calcium and protein nutrition affect bone gain in women in the third decade of life, moderate caffeine intake (one cup of coffee per day, or 103 mg) appears to be safe for bone health in this age group.[22]

HOW LONG DOES CAFFEINE STAY IN YOUR SYSTEM?

In other—more scientific—words, what is the "half-life" of caffeine? Half-life represents the time required for the potency of a substance to fall to half of its initial potency, or to be eliminated from the body. For example, if the amount of a particular drug in your body is 10 of some measure with a half-life of two hours, the amount left in your body after two hours will be 5 of that measure. After that, it drops by half for each subsequent two hours. In general, most healthy individuals of normal weight will eliminate 50 percent of ingested caffeine from their bodies after five to six hours. In a study of normal weight and obese subjects given 162 mg of caffeine orally, the half-life was slightly longer in obese individuals than it was in those of normal weight.[23] The half-life of caffeine tends to be longer as well for women who use birth-control pills.[24] With sustained-release caffeine, you could actually take a lower dose and still feel its benefits without becoming hyperactive. If you are caffeine-sensitive, sustained-release caffeine may be the ideal way to acquire caffeine's benefits minus the annoying side effects.

What makes MSR caffeine the best choice?

Matrix Sustained Release (MSR) caffeine provides balanced energy throughout the day. It gives you a steady level of energy, alertness, and concentration for eight hours in a once-a-day dose. No harsh ups or downs! MSR caffeine also helps stimulate metabolism by mobilizing body fat for fuel and increasing your metabolic rate. All the components of MSR caffeine have been shown to be safe and effective.

Why is the patent number important?

Patents are important for a variety of reasons. The patent of MSR caffeine shows that it is a novel invention based on comprehensive research. It demonstrates that responsible companies will perform the necessary steps to ensure a high-quality product. The authentic form of sustained-release caffeine that has been proven effective in scientific research has been patented to protect products based on it from imitators selling inferior products. So, if you want to get the real benefits of sustained-release caffeine, look for patent number 5,744,164.[25] Otherwise, you'll be paying for a cheap imitation.

A Laundry List
of Benefits

7

s you learned in Chapter 1, caffeine via coffee consumption dates back to the 1400s. Since then, we have had an explosion of caffeine-containing beverages and products—everything from fancy coffees to caffeinated soft drinks and so on. Perhaps the most common reason for consuming caffeine or a caffeinated beverage is its energizing effect. So, whether you are a college student cramming for exams, an office worker suffering from the midday blahs, or an extreme athlete looking for an edge, caffeine just may be the solution for what ails you.

We can thank Dr. David Costill, a prominent exercise physiologist, for his ground-breaking study on caffeine and exercise performance in 1978. His work really put caffeine on the athlete's map. However, in addition to its performance-enhancing and energy-producing benefits, many fitness enthusiasts love caffeine's fat-burning and thermogenic effects. What better way is there to burn fat than to consume caffeine first thing in the morning, and then go to the gym to do your cardiovascular workout? It's easy, it's quick, and it works.

And don't worry about caffeine's safety. After decades of

research, the scientific community has not documented a single firm association between moderate caffeine consumption and any health risk. Using common sense and moderation, the average person can continue to enjoy the benefits of caffeine. Certainly, too much of anything is bad for you. For instance, you can actually overdose on water! But caffeine, used smartly and responsibly, may be the most effective and versatile supplement known.

MSR Caffeine

The authentic form of sustained-release caffeine that has been proven effective by scientific research is patented to protect products based on this technology from imitators selling inferior products. To get the real benefits of sustained-release caffeine, look for patent number 5,744,164.[2] Don't settle for anything less!

Points to Remember

Caffeine (in particular, MSR caffeine):

* Improves performance on tasks that require sustained attention.

* Produces improvement on tasks needing logical reasoning.

* Increases achievement on tasks requiring semantic memory.

* Enhances the absorption of new information.

- Increases the ability to remain alert over a period of time.

- Counteracts the harmful effects of sleep deprivation, as shown on an electroencephalogram (EEG).

- Improves performance of motor actions coming directly from mental activity.

- Increases performance and speed of reaction on a variety of brain-function tests.

- Significantly decreases bodily sway due to fatigue.

- Enhances overall alertness and mental function.

- Decreases the inconsistencies in knowledge that accompany sleep deprivation.

- Increases the body's ability to produce energy by 5 to 15 percent.

- Improves fat burning.

- Raises the metabolic rate in young and old people.

- Elevates metabolism in both lean and obese individuals.

- Further enhances fat burning when taken before exercise.

- Improves endurance during cycling.

- Adds to the pace or effort attainable during exercise.

- Improves muscle strength.

- Lengthens the time to exhaustion.

- Increases the speed possible when swimming sprints.

- Directly affects muscle fibers.

- Does not hinder muscle recovery.

- Extends the benefits without creating the "jitters."

- Has been patented (patent number 5,744,164).[1]

- Is safe and effective.

Notes

Chapter 1

1. http://coffeefaq.com/caffaq.html

2. http://www.benbest.com/health/caffeine.html#chemistry

3. Frary, C.D., R.K. Johnson, and M.Q. Wang. "Food sources and intakes of caffeine in the diets of persons in the United States." *Journal of the American Dietetic Association.* 2005;105(1):110–113.

4. Smith, A.P., R. Clark, and J. Gallagher. "Breakfast cereal and caffeinated coffee: effects on working memory, attention, mood, and cardiovascular function." *Physiology & Behavior.* Aug 1 1999;67(1):9–17.

5. Wesensten, N.J., G. Belenky, D.R. Thorne, et al. "Modafinil vs. caffeine: effects on fatigue during sleep deprivation." *Aviation, Space, and Environmental Medicine.* Jun 2004;75(6):520–525.

6. See note 5 above.

7. van Handel, P.J., E. Burke, D.L. Costill, et al. "Physiological responses to cola ingestion." *Research Quarterly.* May 1977;48(2):436–444.

8. Birnbaum, L.J., and J.D. Herbst. "Physiologic effects of caffeine on cross-country runners." *Journal of Strength and Conditioning Research.* Aug 2004;18(3):463–465.

9. Battram, D.S., J. Shearer, D. Robinson, et al. "Caffeine ingestion does not impede the resynthesis of proglycogen and macroglycogen after prolonged exercise and carbohydrate supplementation in humans." *Journal of Applied Physiology.* Mar 2004;96(3):943–950.

10. Paluska, S.A. "Caffeine and exercise." *Current Sports Medicine Reports.* Aug 2003;2(4):213–219.

11. Motl, R.W., P.J. O'Connor, and R.K. Dishman. "Effect of caffeine on perceptions of leg muscle pain during moderate intensity cycling exercise." *The Journal of Pain.* Aug 2003;4(6):316–321.

12. Jacobs, I., H. Pasternak, and D.G. Bell. "Effects of ephedrine, caffeine, and their combination on muscular endurance." *Medicine and Science in Sports and Exercise.* Jun 2003;35(6):987–994.

13. Davis, J.M., Z. Zhao, H.S. Stock, et al. "Central nervous system effects of caffeine and adenosine on fatigue." *American Journal of Physiology: Regulatory, Integrative and Comparative Physiology.* Feb 2003;284(2):R399–404.

14. Conway, K.J., R. Orr, and S.R. Stannard. "Effect of a divided caffeine dose on endurance cycling performance, postexercise urinary caffeine concentration, and plasma paraxanthine." *Journal of Applied Physiology.* Apr 2003;94(4): 1557–1562.

15. Bell, D.G., and T.M. McLellan. "Effect of repeated caffeine ingestion on repeated exhaustive exercise endurance." *Medicine and Science in Sports and Medicine.* Aug 2003;35(8):1348–1354.

16. Stine, M.M., R.J. O'Connor, B.R. Yatko, et al. "Evidence for a relationship between daily caffeine consumption and accuracy of time estimation." *Human Psychopharmacology.* Oct 2002;17(7):361–367.

17. Hunter, A.M., A. St. Clair Gibson, M. Collins, et al. "Caffeine ingestion does not alter performance during a 100-km cycling time-trial performance." *International Journal of Sport Nutrition and Exercise Metabolism.* Dec 2002;12(4): 438–452.

18. Doherty, M., P.M. Smith, R.C. Davison, et al. "Caffeine is ergogenic after supplementation of oral creatine monohydrate." *Medicine and Science in Sports and Medicine.* Nov 2002;34(11):1785–1792.

19. Cox, G.R., B. Desbrow, P.G. Montgomery, et al. "Effect of different protocols of caffeine intake on metabolism and endurance performance." *Journal of Applied Physiology.* Sep 2002;93(3):990–999.

20. Collomp, K., R. Candau, G. Millet, et al. "Effects of salbutamol and caffeine ingestion on exercise metabolism and performance." *International Journal of Sports Medicine.* Nov 2002;23(8):549–554.

21. Bell, D.G., and T.M. McLellan. "Exercise endurance 1, 3, and 6 h after caffeine ingestion in caffeine users and nonusers." *Journal of Applied Physiology.* Oct 2002;93(4):1227–1234.

22. Armstrong, L.E. "Caffeine, body fluid-electrolyte balance, and exercise performance." *International Journal of Sport Nutrition and Exercise Metabolism.* Jun 2002;12(2):189–206.

23. Cole, K.J., D.L. Costill, R.D. Starling, et al. "Effect of caffeine ingestion on perception of effort and subsequent work production." *International Journal of Sport Nutrition.* Mar 1996;6(1):14–23.

24. Spriet, L.L. "Caffeine and performance." *International Journal of Sport Nutrition.* Jun 1995;5 Suppl:S84–99.

25. Graham, T.E., and L.L. Spriet. "Metabolic, catecholamine, and exercise performance responses to various doses of caffeine." *Journal of Applied Physiology.* Mar 1995;78(3):867–874.

26. Chesley, A., E. Hultman, and L.L. Spriet. "Effects of epinephrine infusion on muscle glycogenolysis during intense aerobic exercise." *The American Journal of Physiology.* Jan 1995;268(1 Pt 1):E127–134.

27. Van Soeren, M.H., P. Sathasivam, L.L. Spriet, et al. "Caffeine metabolism and epinephrine responses during exercise in users and nonusers." *Journal of Applied Physiology.* Aug 1993;75(2):805–812.

28. Lindinger, M.I., T.E. Graham, and L.L. Spriet. "Caffeine attenuates the exercise-induced increase in plasma [K+] in humans." *Journal of Applied Physiology.* Mar 1993;74(3):1149–1155.

29. Spriet, L.L., D.A. MacLean, D.J. Dyck, et al. "Caffeine ingestion and muscle metabolism during prolonged exercise in humans." *The American Journal of Physiology.* Jun 1992;262(6 Pt 1):E891–898.

30. Collomp, K., S. Ahmaidi, J.C. Chatard, et al. "Benefits of caffeine ingestion on sprint performance in trained and untrained swimmers." *European Journal of Applied Physiology and Occupational Physiology.* 1992;64(4):377–380.

31. Anselme, F., K. Collomp, B. Mercier, et al. "Caffeine increases maximal anaerobic power and blood lactate concentration." *European Journal of Applied Physiology and Occupational Physiology.* 1992;65(2):188–191.

32. Collomp, K., S. Ahmaidi, M. Audran, et al. "Effects of caffeine ingestion on performance and anaerobic metabolism during the Wingate Test." *International Journal of Sports Medicine.* Oct 1991;12(5):439–443.

33. Collomp, K., F. Anselme, M. Audran, et al. Effects of moderate exercise on the pharmacokinetics of caffeine. *European Journal of Clinical Pharmacology.* 1991;40(3):279–282.

34. Erickson, M.A., R.J. Schwarzkopf, and R.D. McKenzie. "Effects of caffeine, fructose, and glucose ingestion on muscle glycogen utilization during exercise." *Medicine and Science in Sports and Medicine.* Dec 1987;19(6):579–583.

35. Nassar-Gentina, V., J.V. Passonneau, and S.I. Rapoport. "Fatigue and metabolism of frog muscle fibers during stimulation and in response to caffeine." *The American Journal of Physiology.* Sep 1981;241(3):C160–166.

36. Ivy, J.L., D.L. Costill, W.J. Fink, et al. "Influence of caffeine and carbohydrate feedings on endurance performance." *Medicine and Science in Sports.* Spring 1979;11(1):6–11.

37. Costill, D.L., G.P. Dalsky, and W.J. Fink. "Effects of caffeine ingestion on metabolism and exercise performance." *Medicine and Science in Sports.* Fall 1978;10(3):155–158.

38. See note 37 above.

39. Zahorska-Markiewicz, B. "[Does post-caffeine increase in thermogenesis facilitate the treatment of obesity?]" *Polski Tygodnik Lekarski (Warsaw, Poland).* May 12 1980;35(19):697–699.

40. Acheson, K.J., G. Gremaud, I. Meirim, et al. "Metabolic effects of caffeine in humans: lipid oxidation or futile cycling?" *The American Journal of Clinical Nutrition.* Jan 2004;79(1):40–46.

41. Ryu, S., S.K. Choi, S.S. Joung, et al. "Caffeine as a lipolytic food component increases endurance performance in rats and athletes." *Journal of Nutritional Science and Vitaminology (Tokyo, Japan).* Apr 2001;47(2):139–146.

42. Arciero, P.J., C.L. Bougopoulos, B.C. Nindl, et al. "Influence of age on the thermic response to caffeine in women." *Metabolism.* Jan 2000;49(1):101–107.

43. Jiang, M., K. Kameda, L.K. Han, et al. "Isolation of lipolytic substances caffeine and 1,7-dimethylxanthine from the stem and rhizome of Sinomenium actum." *Planta Medica.* May 1998;64(4):375–377.

44. Koot, P., and P. Deurenberg. "Comparison of changes in energy expenditure and body temperatures after caffeine consumption." *Annals of Nutrition & Metabolism.* 1995;39(3):135–142.

45. Bracco, D., J.M. Ferrarra, M.J. Arnaud, et al. "Effects of caffeine on energy metabolism, heart rate, and methylxanthine metabolism in lean and obese women." *The American Journal of Physiology.* Oct 1995;269(4 Pt 1):E671–678.

46. Arciero, P.J., A.W. Gardner, J. Calles-Escandon, et al. "Effects of caffeine ingestion on NE kinetics, fat oxidation, and energy expenditure in younger and older men." *The American Journal of Physiology.* Jun 1995;268(6 Pt 1):E1192–1198.

47. Zhang, Y., and J.N. Wells. "The effects of chronic caffeine administration on peripheral adenosine receptors." *The Journal of Pharmacology and Experimental Therapeutics.* Sep 1990;254(3):757–763.

48. Hetzler, R.K., R.G. Knowlton, S.M. Somani, et al. "Effect of paraxanthine on FFA mobilization after intravenous caffeine administration in humans." *Journal of Applied Physiology.* Jan 1990;68(1):44–47.

49. Astrup, A., S. Toubro, S. Cannon, et al. "Caffeine: a double-blind, placebo-controlled study of its thermogenic, metabolic, and cardiovascular effects in healthy volunteers." *The American Journal of Clinical Nutrition.* May 1990;51(5): 759–767.

50. Dulloo, A.G., C.A. Geissler, T. Horton, et al. "Normal caffeine consumption: influence on thermogenesis and daily energy expenditure in lean and post obese human volunteers." *The American Journal of Clinical Nutrition.* Jan 1989;49(1):44–50.

51. Cheung, W.T., C.M. Lee, and T.B. Ng. "Potentiation of the anti-lipolytic effect of 2-chloroadenosine after chronic caffeine treatment." *Pharmacology.* 1988;36(5):331–339.

52. Powers, S.K., and S. Dodd. "Caffeine and endurance performance." *Sports Medicine (Auckland, Australia).* May-Jun 1985;2(3):165–174.

53. Poehlman, E.T., J.P. Despres, H. Bessette, et al. "Influence of caffeine on the resting metabolic rate of exercise-trained and inactive subjects." *Medicine and Science in Sports and Exercise.* Dec 1985;17(6):689–694.

54. Izawa, T., E. Koshimizu, T. Komabayashi, et al. "[Effects of Ca2+ and calmodulin inhibitors on lipolysis induced by epinephrine, norepinephrine, caffeine and ACTH in rat epididymal adipose tissue]." *Nippon Seirigaku Zasshi: Journal of the Physiological Society of Japan.* 1983;45(1):36–44.

55. See note 46 above.

56. Nawrot, P., S. Jordan, J. Eastwood, et al. "Effects of caffeine on human health." *Food Additives and Contaminants.* Jan 2003;20(1):1–30.

57. Chou, T.M., and N.L. Benowitz. "Caffeine and coffee: effects on health and cardiovascular disease." *Comparative Biochemistry and Physiology: Part C, Pharmacology, Toxicology & Endocrinology.* Oct 1994;109(2):173–189.

58. Agardh, E.E., S. Carlsson, A. Ahlbom, et al. "Coffee consumption, type 2 diabetes and impaired glucose tolerance in Swedish men and women." *Journal of Internal Medicine*. Jun 2004;255(6):645–652.

59. Michels, K.B., L. Holmberg, L. Bergkvist, et al. "Coffee, tea, and caffeine consumption and breast cancer incidence in a cohort of Swedish women." *Annals of Epidemiology*. Jan 2002;12(1):21–26.

60. Heaney, R.P. "Effects of caffeine on bone and the calcium economy." *Chemical Toxicology*. 2002;40(9):1263–1270.

61. Packard, P.T., and R.R. Recker. "Caffeine does not affect the rate of gain in spine bone in young women." *Osteoporosis International*. 1996;6(2):149–152.

62. Forbes, J.A., K.F. Jones, C.J. Kehm, et al. "Evaluation of aspirin, caffeine, and their combination in postoperative oral surgery pain." *Pharmacotherapy*. 1990;10(6):387–393.

63. Goldstein, J., H.D. Hoffman, J.J. Armellino, et al. "Treatment of severe, disabling migraine attacks in an over-the-counter population of migraine sufferers: results from three randomized, placebo-controlled studies of the combination of acetaminophen, aspirin, and caffeine." *Cephalalgia: An International Journal of Headache*. Sep 1999;19(7):684–691.

64. Peroutka, S.J., J.A. Lyon, J. Swarbrick, et al. "Efficacy of diclofenac sodium soft gel 100 mg with or without caffeine 100 mg in migraine without aura: a randomized, double-blind, crossover study." *Headache*. Feb 2004;44(2):136–141.

65. See notes 62–64 above.

Chapter 2

1. Paluska, S.A. "Caffeine and exercise." *Current Sports Medicine Reports*. Aug 2003;2(4):213–219.

2. Bell, D.G., and T.M. McLellan. "Effect of repeated caffeine ingestion on repeated exhaustive exercise endurance." *Medicine and Science in Sports and Medicine*. Aug 2003;35(8):1348–1354.

3. Stine, M.M., R.J. O'Connor, B.R. Yatko, et al. "Evidence for a relationship between daily caffeine consumption and accuracy of time estimation." *Human Psychopharmacology*. Oct 2002;17(7):361–367.

4. Doherty, M., P.M. Smith, R.C. Davison, et al. "Caffeine is ergogenic after supplementation of oral creatine monohydrate." *Medicine and Science in Sports and Medicine*. Nov 2002;34(11):1785–1792.

5. Cox, G.R., B. Desbrow, P.G. Montgomery, et al. "Effect of different pro-tocols of caffeine intake on metabolism and endurance performance." *Journal of Applied Physiology.* Sep 2002;93(3):990–999.

6. Chauffard, F., M.Y.A. Enslen, and P. Tachon. "Sustained release micro-particulate caffeine formulation." U.S. Patent 5,744,164. April 28, 1998. http://patft.uspto.gov/netacgi/nph-Parser?Sect1=PTO1&Sect2=HITOFF &d=PALL&p=1&u=/netahtml/srchnum.htm&r=1&f=G&l=50&s1=5,744 ,164.WKU.&OS=PN/5,744,164&RS=PN/5,744,164.

7. Patat, A., P. Rosenzweig, M. Enslen, et al. "Effects of a new slow release formulation of caffeine on EEG, psychomotor and cognitive functions in sleep-deprived subjects." *Human Psychopharmacology.* Apr 2000;15(3): 153–170.

8. Beaumont, M., D. Batejat, C. Pierard, et al. "Slow release caffeine and prolonged (64-h) continuous wakefulness: effects on vigilance and cogni-tive performance." *Journal of Sleep Research.* Dec 2001;10(4):265–276.

9. Pierard, C., M. Beaumont, M. Enslen, et al. "Resynchronization of hor-monal rhythms after an eastbound flight in humans: effects of slow-release caffeine and melatonin." *European Journal of Applied Physiology.* Jul 2001;85(1-2):144–150.

10. Acheson, K.J., G. Gremaud, I. Meirim, et al. "Metabolic effects of caf-feine in humans: lipid oxidation or futile cycling?" *The American Journal of Clinical Nutrition.* Jan 2004;79(1):40–46.

11. Zahorska-Markiewicz, B. "[Does post-caffeine increase in thermogen-esis facilitate the treatment of obesity?]" *Polski Tygodnik Lekarski* (*Warsaw, Poland*). May 12 1980;35(19):697–699.

Chapter 3

1. McLellan, T.M., D.G. Bell, and G.H. Kamimori. "Caffeine improves physical performance during 24 h of active wakefulness." *Aviation, Space, and Environmental Medicine.* Aug 2004;75(8):666–672.

2. See note 1 above.

3. Patat, A., P. Rosenzweig, M. Enslen, et al. "Effects of a new slow release formulation of caffeine on EEG, psychomotor and cognitive functions in sleep-deprived subjects." *Human Psychopharmacology.* Apr 2000;15(3): 153–170.

4. Beaumont, M., D. Batejat, C. Pierard, et al. "Slow release caffeine and prolonged (64-h) continuous wakefulness: effects on vigilance and cogni-tive performance." *Journal of Sleep Research.* Dec 2001;10(4):265–276.

5. Smith, A.P., R. Clark, and J. Gallagher. "Breakfast cereal and caffeinated coffee: effects on working memory, attention, mood, and cardiovascular function." *Physiology & Behavior*. Aug 1 1999;67(1):9–17.

6. Tikuisis, P., A.A. Keefe, T.M. McLellan, et al. "Caffeine restores engagement speed but not shooting precision following 22 h of active wakefulness." *Aviation, Space, and Environmental Medicine*. Sep 2004;75(9):771–776.

7. Robelin, M., and P.J. Rogers. "Mood and psychomotor performance effects of the first, but not of subsequent, cup-of-coffee equivalent doses of caffeine consumed after overnight caffeine abstinence." *Behavioural Pharmacology*. Nov 1998;9(7):611–618.

8. Reyner, L.A., and J.A. Horne. "Early morning driver sleepiness: effectiveness of 200 mg caffeine." *Psychophysiology*. Mar 2000;37(2):251–256.

9. Jarvis, M.J. "Does caffeine intake enhance absolute levels of cognitive performance?" *Psychopharmacology (Berl)*. 1993;110(1-2):45–52.

Chapter 4

1. Battram, D.S., J. Shearer, D. Robinson, et al. "Caffeine ingestion does not impede the resynthesis of proglycogen and macroglycogen after prolonged exercise and carbohydrate supplementation in humans." *Journal of Applied Physiology*. Mar 2004;96(3):943–950.

2. Paluska, S.A. "Caffeine and exercise." *Current Sports Medicine Reports*. Aug 2003;2(4):213–219.

3. Motl, R.W., P.J. O'Connor, and R.K. Dishman. "Effect of caffeine on perceptions of leg muscle pain during moderate intensity cycling exercise." *The Journal of Pain*. Aug 2003;4(6):316–321.

4. Jacobs, I., H. Pasternak, and D.G. Bell. "Effects of ephedrine, caffeine, and their combination on muscular endurance." *Medicine and Science in Sports and Exercise*. Jun 2003;35(6):987–994.

5. Davis, J.M., Z. Zhao, H.S. Stock, et al. "Central nervous system effects of caffeine and adenosine on fatigue." *American Journal of Physiology: Regulatory, Integrative and Comparative Physiology*. Feb 2003;284(2): R399–404.

6. Conway, K.J., R. Orr, and S.R. Stannard. "Effect of a divided caffeine dose on endurance cycling performance, postexercise urinary caffeine concentration, and plasma paraxanthine." *Journal of Applied Physiology*. Apr 2003;94(4): 1557–1562.

7. Bell, D.G., and T.M. McLellan. "Effect of repeated caffeine ingestion on repeated exhaustive exercise endurance." *Medicine and Science in Sports and Medicine.* Aug 2003;35(8):1348–1354.

8. Stine, M.M., R.J. O'Connor, B.R. Yatko, et al. "Evidence for a relationship between daily caffeine consumption and accuracy of time estimation." *Human Psychopharmacology.* Oct 2002;17(7):361–367.

9. Doherty, M., P.M. Smith, R.C. Davison, et al. "Caffeine is ergogenic after supplementation of oral creatine monohydrate." *Medicine and Science in Sports and Medicine.* Nov 2002;34(11):1785–1792.

10. Cox, G.R., B. Desbrow, P.G. Montgomery, et al. "Effect of different protocols of caffeine intake on metabolism and endurance performance." *Journal of Applied Physiology.* Sep 2002;93(3):990–999.

11. Bell, D.G., and T.M. McLellan. "Exercise endurance 1, 3, and 6 h after caffeine ingestion in caffeine users and nonusers." *Journal of Applied Physiology.* Oct 2002;93(4):1227–1234.

12. Armstrong, L.E. "Caffeine, body fluid-electrolyte balance, and exercise performance." *International Journal of Sport Nutrition and Exercise Metabolism.* Jun 2002;12(2):189–206.

13. Cole, K.J., D.L. Costill, R.D. Starling, et al. "Effect of caffeine ingestion on perception of effort and subsequent work production." *International Journal of Sport Nutrition.* Mar 1996;6(1):14–23.

14. Spriet, L.L. "Caffeine and performance." *International Journal of Sport Nutrition.* Jun 1995;5 Suppl:S84–99.

15. Graham, T.E., and L.L. Spriet. "Metabolic, catecholamine, and exercise performance responses to various doses of caffeine." *Journal of Applied Physiology.* Mar 1995;78(3):867–874.

16. Chesley, A., E. Hultman, and L.L. Spriet. "Effects of epinephrine infusion on muscle glycogenolysis during intense aerobic exercise." *The American Journal of Physiology.* Jan 1995;268(1 Pt 1):E127–134.

17. Van Soeren, M.H., P. Sathasivam, L.L. Spriet, et al. "Caffeine metabolism and epinephrine responses during exercise in users and nonusers." *Journal of Applied Physiology.* Aug 1993;75(2):805–812.

18. Lindinger, M.I., T.E. Graham, and L.L. Spriet. "Caffeine attenuates the exercise-induced increase in plasma [K+] in humans." *Journal of Applied Physiology.* Mar 1993;74(3):1149–1155.

19. Spriet, L.L., D.A. MacLean, D.J. Dyck, et al. "Caffeine ingestion and muscle metabolism during prolonged exercise in humans." *The American Journal of Physiology.* Jun 1992;262(6 Pt 1):E891–898.

20. Collomp, K., S. Ahmaidi, J.C. Chatard, et al. "Benefits of caffeine ingestion on sprint performance in trained and untrained swimmers." *European Journal of Applied Physiology and Occupational Physiology.* 1992; 64(4):377–380.

21. Anselme, F., K. Collomp, B. Mercier, et al. "Caffeine increases maximal anaerobic power and blood lactate concentration." *European Journal of Applied Physiology and Occupational Physiology.* 1992;65(2):188–191.

22. Collomp, K., S. Ahmaidi, M. Audran, et al. "Effects of caffeine ingestion on performance and anaerobic metabolism during the Wingate Test." *International Journal of Sports Medicine.* Oct 1991;12(5):439–443.

23. Collomp, K., F. Anselme, M. Audran, et al. "Effects of moderate exercise on the pharmacokinetics of caffeine." *European Journal of Clinical Pharmacology.* 1991;40(3):279–282.

24. Ivy, J.L., D.L. Costill, W.J. Fink, et al. "Influence of caffeine and carbohydrate feedings on endurance performance." *Medicine and Science in Sports.* Spring 1979;11(1):6–11.

25. Costill, D.L., G.P. Dalsky, and W.J. Fink. "Effects of caffeine ingestion on metabolism and exercise performance." *Medicine and Science in Sports.* Fall 1978;10(3):155–158.

26. Zahorska-Markiewicz, B. "[Does post-caffeine increase in thermogenesis facilitate the treatment of obesity?]" *Polski Tygodnik Lekarski (Warsaw, Poland).* May 12 1980;35(19):697–699.

27. See note 20 above.

28. See note 8 above.

29. Acheson, K.J., G. Gremaud, I. Meirim, et al. "Metabolic effects of caffeine in humans: lipid oxidation or futile cycling?" *The American Journal of Clinical Nutrition.* Jan 2004;79(1):40–46.

30. Jacobson, B.H., M.D. Weber, L. Claypool, et al. "Effect of caffeine on maximal strength and power in elite male athletes." *British Journal of Sports Medicine.* Dec 1992;26(4):276–280.

31. See note 20 above.

32. Strong, F.C., 3rd. "It may be the caffeine in Extra Strength Excedrin

that is effective for migraine." *The Journal of Pharmacy and Pharmacology.* Dec 1997; 49(12):1260.

33. See note 9 above.

34. O'Connor, P.J., R.W. Motl, S.P. Broglio, et al. "Dose-dependent effect of caffeine on reducing leg muscle pain during cycling exercise is unrelated to systolic blood pressure." *Pain.* Jun 2004;109(3):291–298. See also note 3 above.

35. Tarnopolsky, M., and C. Cupido. "Caffeine potentiates low frequency skeletal muscle force in habitual and nonhabitual caffeine consumers." *Journal of Applied Physiology.* Nov 2000;89(5):1719–1724.

Chapter 5

1. Dulloo, A.G., C.A. Geissler, T. Horton, et al. "Normal caffeine consumption: influence on thermogenesis and daily energy expenditure in lean and post obese human volunteers." *The American Journal of Clinical Nutrition.* Jan 1989;49(1):44–50.

2. Astrup, A., S. Toubro, S. Cannon, et al. "Caffeine: a double-blind, placebo-controlled study of its thermogenic, metabolic, and cardiovascular effects in healthy volunteers." *The American Journal of Clinical Nutrition.* May 1990;51 (5):759–767.

3. Poehlman, E.T., J.P. Despres, H. Bessette, et al. "Influence of caffeine on the resting metabolic rate of exercise-trained and inactive subjects." *Medicine and Science in Sports and Exercise.* Dec 1985;17(6):689–694.

4. See note 1 above.

5. Arciero, P.J., A.W. Gardner, J. Calles-Escandon, et al. "Effects of caffeine ingestion on NE kinetics, fat oxidation, and energy expenditure in younger and older men." *The American Journal of Physiology.* Jun 1995; 268(6 Pt 1): E1192–1198.

6. Koot, P., and P. Deurenberg. "Comparison of changes in energy expenditure and body temperatures after caffeine consumption." *Annals of Nutrition & Metabolism.* 1995;39(3):135–142. See also note 5.

7. Acheson, K.J., G. Gremaud, I. Meirim, et al. "Metabolic effects of caffeine in humans: lipid oxidation or futile cycling?" *The American Journal of Clinical Nutrition.* Jan 2004;79(1):40–46.

8. Bracco, D., J.M. Ferrarra, M.J. Arnaud, et al. "Effects of caffeine on energy metabolism, heart rate, and methylxanthine metabolism in lean and

obese women." *The American Journal of Physiology*. Oct 1995;269(4 Pt 1):E671–678.

9. Acheson, K.J., B. Zahorska-Markiewicz, P. Pittet, et al. "Caffeine and coffee: their influence on metabolic rate and substrate utilization in normal weight and obese individuals." *The American Journal of Clinical Nutrition*. May 1980;33 (5):989–997.

10. Jung, R.T., P.S. Shetty, W.P. James, et al. "Caffeine: its effect on catecholamines and metabolism in lean and obese humans." *Clinical Science (London, England)*. May 1981;60(5):527–535.

11. See note 1 above.

Chapter 6

1. Forbes, J.A., K.F. Jones, C.J. Kehm, et al. "Evaluation of aspirin, caffeine, and their combination in postoperative oral surgery pain." *Pharmacotherapy*. 1990;10(6):387–393.

2. Goldstein, J., H.D. Hoffman, J.J. Armellino, et al. "Treatment of severe, disabling migraine attacks in an over-the-counter population of migraine sufferers: results from three randomized, placebo-controlled studies of the combination of acetaminophen, aspirin, and caffeine." *Cephalalgia: An International Journal of Headache*. Sep 1999;19(7):684–691.

3. Peroutka, S.J., J.A. Lyon, J. Swarbrick, et al. "Efficacy of diclofenac sodium soft gel 100 mg with or without caffeine 100 mg in migraine without aura: a randomized, double-blind, crossover study." *Headache*. Feb 2004; 44(2):136–141.

4. See notes 1–3 above.

5. Wrenn, K.D., I. Oschner. "Rhabdomyolysis induced by a caffeine overdose." *Annals of Emergency Medicine*. Jan 1989;18(1):94–97.

6. http://www.extension.umn.edu/info-u/nutrition/BJ884.html; http://coffeefaq.com/caffaq.html

7. Bracken, M.B., E.W. Triche, K. Belanger, et al. "Association of maternal caffeine consumption with decrements in fetal growth." *American Journal of Epidemiology*. Mar 1 2003;157(5):456–466.

8. Vik, T., L.S. Bakketeig, K.U. Trygg, et al. "High caffeine consumption in the third trimester of pregnancy: gender-specific effects on fetal growth." *Paediatric and Perinatal Epidemiology*. Oct 2003;17(4):324–331.

9. Tolstrup, J.S., S.K. Kjaer, C. Munk, et al. "Does caffeine and alcohol

intake before pregnancy predict the occurrence of spontaneous abortion?" *Human Reproduction (Oxford, England)*. Dec 2003;18(12):2704–2710.

10. Castellanos, F.X., and J.L. Rapoport. "Effects of caffeine on development and behavior in infancy and childhood: a review of the published literature." *Food and Chemical Toxicology*. Sep 2002;40(9):1235–1242.

11. Hering-Hanit, R., and N. Gadoth. "Caffeine-induced headache in children and adolescents." *Cephalalgia: An International Journal of Headache*. Jun 2003; 23(5):332–335.

12. Nawrot, P., S. Jordan, J. Eastwood, et al. "Effects of caffeine on human health." *Food Additives and Contaminants*. Jan 2003;20(1):1–30.

13. Nehlig, A., and S. Boyet. "Dose-response study of caffeine effects on cerebral functional activity with a specific focus on dependence." *Brain Research*. Mar 6 2000;858(1):71–77.

14. Chou, T.M., and N.L. Benowitz. "Caffeine and coffee: effects on health and cardiovascular disease." *Comparative Biochemistry and Physiology: Part C, Pharmacology, Toxicology & Endocrinology*. Oct 1994;109(2):173–189.

15. Salazar-Martinez, E., W.C. Willett, A. Ascherio, et al. "Coffee consumption and risk for type 2 diabetes mellitus." *Annals of Internal Medicine*. Jan 6 2004;140(1):1–8.

16. Agardh, E.E., S. Carlsson, A. Ahlbom, et al. "Coffee consumption, type 2 diabetes and impaired glucose tolerance in Swedish men and women." *Journal of Internal Medicine*. Jun 2004;255(6):645–652.

17. Michels, K.B., L. Holmberg, L. Bergkvist, et al. "Coffee, tea, and caffeine consumption and breast cancer incidence in a cohort of Swedish women." *Annals of Epidemiology*. Jan 2002;12(1):21–26.

18. Marshall, J., S. Graham, and M. Swanson. "Caffeine consumption and benign breast disease: a case-control comparison." *American Journal of Public Health*. Jun 1982;72(6):610–612.

19. Lou, Y.R., Y.P. Lu, J.G. Xie, et al. "Effects of oral administration of tea, decaffeinated tea, and caffeine on the formation and growth of tumors in high-risk SKH-1 mice previously treated with ultraviolet B light." *Nutrition and Cancer*. 1999;33(2):146–153.

20. Heaney, R.P. "Effects of caffeine on bone and the calcium economy." *Chemical Toxicology*. 2002;40(9):1263–1270.

21. See note 20 above.

22. Packard, P.T., and R.R. Recker. "Caffeine does not affect the rate of

gain in spine bone in young women." *Osteoporosis International.* 1996;6(2):149–152.

23. Abernethy, D.R., E.L. Todd, and J.B. Schwartz. "Caffeine disposition in obesity." *British Journal of Clinical Pharmacology.* 1985;20(1):61–66.

24. Abernethy, D.R., and E.L. Todd. "Impairment of caffeine clearance by chronic use of low-dose oestrogen-containing oral contraceptives." *European Journal of Clinical Pharmacology.* 1985;28(4):425–428.

25. Chauffard, F., M.Y.A. Enslen, and P. Tachon. "Sustained release microparticulate caffeine formulation." U.S. Patent 5,744,164. April 28, 1998. http://patft.uspto.gov/netacgi/nph-Parser?Sect1=PTO1&Sect2=HITOFF &d=PALL&p=1&u=/netahtml/srchnum.htm&r=1&f=G&l=50&s1=5,744 ,164.WKU.&OS=PN/5,744,164&RS=PN/5,744,164.

Chapter 7

1. Chauffard, F., M.Y.A. Enslen, and P. Tachon. "Sustained release microparticulate caffeine formulation." U.S. Patent 5,744,164. April 28, 1998. http://patft.uspto.gov/netacgi/nph-Parser?Sect1=PTO1&Sect2=HITOFF &d=PALL&p=1&u=/netahtml/srchnum.htm&r=1&f=G&l=50&s1=5,744 ,164.WKU.&OS=PN/5,744,164&RS=PN/5,744,164.

2. See note 1 above.

Index

A

Accidents, sleep-related, 25–26
Adenosine triphosphate, 8
American Journal of Clinical Nutrition, The, 17
ATP. *See* Adenosine triphosphate.

B

Blood pressure, caffeine and, 41
Bone health, caffeine and, 9, 50
Brain Research, 48
Breakfast with caffeine, 24
Breast cancer, caffeine and. *See* Cancer, caffeine and.

C

Caffeine
   addictiveness of, 48
   age and, 6–7
   benefits of, 1. *See also* Energy; Performance Enhancement; Thermogenesis.
   brain function and, 23
   chemical structure of, 2
   consumption. *See* Caffeine intake.
   creatine and, 12
   half-life of, 50–51
   main sources of, 3
   method of action, 37
   moderate intake, 45
   NSAIDs and, 45
   pain relief and, 9
   points to remember (*complete*), 54–56
   regular, drawbacks of, 12
   safety of, 8–9
   sustained-release. *See* Sustained-release caffeine.

About the Author

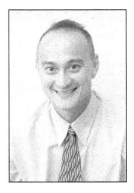 **Jose Antonio, Ph.D., C.S.C.S., F.A.C.S.M.,** is a leading research advocate in the field of performance nutrition. He is the chief executive officer of the International Society of Sports Nutrition (www. sportsnutritionsociety.org), the only academic society dedicated to promoting the science and practice of sports nutrition. Currently, he is the chief science officer of Javalution Coffee Company (www. javalution.com), consultant to the Specialty Nutrition Group (www. specialtynutrition.com), and sports nutrition editor for *AXL Magazine.*

Dr. Antonio is a prolific writer and speaker in the field of sports and performance nutrition, and a popular consultant to the industry. He has published more than forty peer-reviewed scientific papers and has written six books in the field of sports nutrition and exercise (www.joseantoniophd.com). Dr. Antonio earned a Ph.D. and completed a postdoctoral fellowship at the University of Texas Southwestern Medical Center in Dallas.

Printed in the USA
CPSIA information can be obtained
at www.ICGtesting.com
JSHW012009140824
68134JS00004B/94

9 781681 627878